THE
Resilient
Nurse
BOOK

A NURSE'S GUIDE TO BUILDING INNER STRENGTH
WHEN HELPING OTHERS IS HURTING YOU

Karen F. Furr

Published in Denver, Colorado, by Paper Raven Books.

This title may be purchased in bulk for education or business use. For information, please email karen@rnproject.org

Scripture taken from the Holy Bible, *New International Version®*, *NIV®*. Copyright © 1973, 1978, 1984 by Biblica, Inc.™ Used by permission of Zondervan. All rights reserved worldwide.

Printed in the United States of America

First Printing, 2022

ISBN 979-8-9857606-2-0 (Paperback edition)
ISBN 979-8-9857606-3-7 (Hardback edition)

Art by Lauren Morris

"You can't decide if *you get through this,*
but you can decide how *you get through this."*

— Steve Fowler (Dad)

FREE BONUS

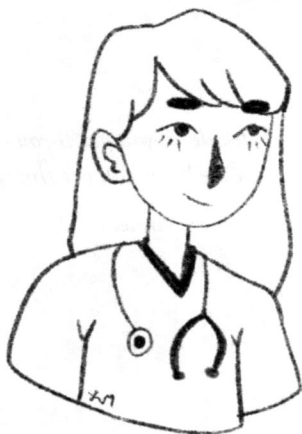

What's Your Resilience Personality?

Scan the QR code to discover your resilience personality and what that means for you as a nurse.

Contents

Contents

DEDICATION

*This book is dedicated to my mom,
the most intelligent, caring, resilient nurse I know.*

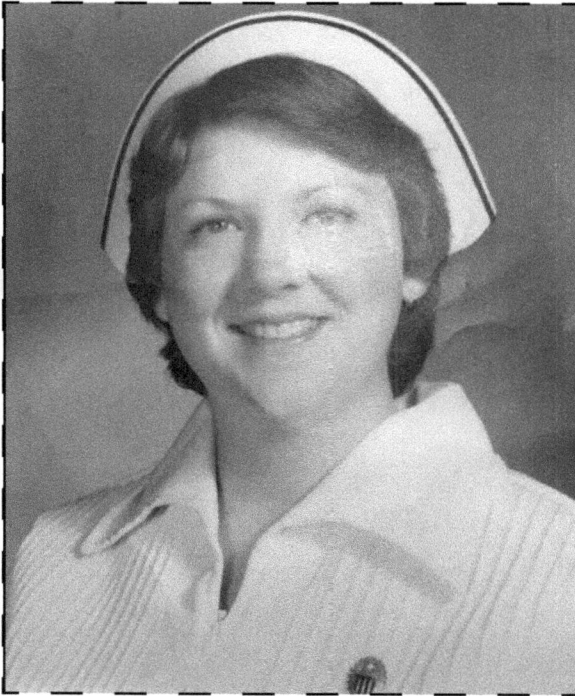

*Janice M. Fowler
St. Mary's School of Nursing
Class of 1977*

GIVING CREDIT
WHERE CREDIT IS DUE

Perhaps the most profound influence in the creation of The Resilient Nurse Project was the book *Stronger*, by George Everly Jr., Dr. Douglas Strouse, and Dr. Dennis K. McCormack.[1] In 2018, I participated in a class offered by my employer at the time, in which we read this book and then came together to review the lessons as they applied to our various jobs in the pediatric hospital system. I began to apply these principles to my own life and work as a nurse, and it immediately made sense. I then began to talk to colleagues and fellow nurses about their resilience practices, self-care strategies, and coping mechanisms. This book, along with the additional information I learned from my informal research of surveying and chatting with hundreds of nurses, led me to develop the foundation upon which The Resilient Nurse Project is built.

In their book, Everly, Strouse, and McCormack describe what they term "five factors of personal resilience." Those factors are active optimism, decisive action, moral compass, relentless

---

1 George Everly, Jr., Douglas Strouse, and Dennis McCormack, *Stronger: Develop the Resilience You Need to Succeed* (New York: Amacom, 2015).

tenacity, and interpersonal support. It was in my ongoing dialogue with colleagues that I found nurses tend to apply one additional "category" not specifically described in the book: intentional self-care. I want to be clear that these ideas were not originated by me but rather learned and applied to the profession of nursing in my work with The Resilient Nurse Project. Everly, Strouse, and McCormack deserve all the credit for the work they laid out, and the nurses who allowed me to ask questions and share their stories and struggles deserve all that can be learned from that work.

INTRODUCTION

I grew up in a home of givers.

My mom was a nurse, my dad was a firefighter, and the selfless characteristics required by those careers define their personalities to the core, even though they are both retired now.

When I unexpectedly found myself in the tough position of being a single mom with a toddler and another baby on the way, I knew nursing would be the best career for me to support my children. So, I worked hard and earned my bachelor's degree in the field.

I started my career as a nurse in a Pediatric Intensive Care Unit (PICU) and loved it! But it only took a few years for me to start feeling overwhelmed, stressed, and burned out. Since everyone else around me expressed the same feelings, I assumed this was just "part of the job" and tried to accept it.

Then 2014 came, and my youngest daughter (nine years old at the time) was diagnosed with brain cancer. I quickly realized that I was already so emotionally, mentally, and physically "spent" from caring for other people's sick children that I barely had anything left to give her. This desperation led me to research ways that I could give my best to her and my family. (Thankfully, she received excellent care and treatment and is now seven years in remission!)

But I just couldn't shake the feeling that "nursing" shouldn't be this way. I wanted to somehow make a difference and help nurses find better ways to deal with the stresses of their careers. In 2019, I earned my master's degree in nursing education and decided to teach nurses how to thrive in their careers without feeling like they have to sacrifice in other parts of their lives.

And so The Resilient Nurse Project was born.

Our mission is to help nurses recognize, address, and overcome burnout and compassion fatigue. When the mounting pressures that nurses face were exposed and compounded by the COVID pandemic, I realized that this message needed to be shared more than ever before. Someone needs to help "heal the healer" and advocate for nurses while they are so busy advocating for their patients. That "someone" is ME!

But it's not all about me. I'm just one of 4.2 million registered nurses in the United States, according to the *Journal of Nursing Regulation*'s 2020 National Nursing Workforce Survey.[2] In addition, there are 950,000 licensed practical/vocational nurses.

This book will share the six pillars of resilience that I learned from my research and conversations with nurses, which became the foundation of everything we teach at The Resilient Nurse Project. Essentially, these are six different areas that we can strengthen in ourselves, which will build a toolkit of resilience and strength. Then, no matter what situation we face, we can pull from one of the six pillars to cope. When we equip our subconscious with all of these tools, then we learn to pull from whichever one we need depending on the situation or crisis we face.

Many nurses I talk to have one pillar of resilience—one coping mechanism they rely on when they become stressed or overwhelmed or have a bad day. And that's ok when life

---

2 Richard A. Smiley, et al., "The 2020 National Nursing Workforce Survey," *Journal of Nursing Regulation* 12, no. 1 (2021), https://doi.org/10.1016/S2155-8256(21)00027-2.

circumstances are fairly normal, and little bumps come along. But when a stressor hits on a totally new level, that one pillar is no longer enough. When we don't have anything else to pull from or dig deeper into for help, feelings of overwhelm and defeat occur. When we build a full, comprehensive toolkit of resilience, we have whatever we need, regardless of the situation.

In addition, this book will serve as an avenue for other nurses to share their own stories of how they relied on these pillars of resilience to overcome their unique challenges.

At The Resilient Nurse Project, we develop each of these pillars so they can work together. When I'm working individually with a nurse coaching client, we start by ranking the pillars from strongest to weakest, as they relate to that person, and then we talk about one pillar at a time, learning personalized approaches to strengthen that pillar so that the nurse has more tools from which to pull.

When we practice these regularly, we allow our subconscious to file them away as options to call upon when the rubber hits the road. When we identify ways to implement these different resilience pillars, when the stress starts to build up, our mind automatically pulls from these categories and balances the different areas so we have a multitude of strengths working for us. It allows us to serve and care for others without completely depleting ourselves.

The application of the six pillars of resilience employs a holistic approach that teaches us to listen to our body and environment, be mindful to bring our full attention to each situation, and then select the right tool for that moment.

ACTIVE OPTIMISM

Optimism can be described as seeing the world from a "glass half full" perspective. It's seeing the silver lining, the positive in any given situation or circumstance. The key to "active optimism" is the "active" part. People who practice active optimism choose to take steps to increase the chances of a positive outcome, instead of just waiting to see what happens.

Optimism doesn't come naturally for most of us. Our amygdala is constantly processing our surroundings for threats and potential danger, so it's no wonder we notice the negative first. But we can learn how to also recognize the positive potential in our environment. And we all know that a positive mood leads to positive energy, leading to positive relationships, and so forth.

In her book, *The How of Happiness,* Sonja Lyubomirsky says, "All that is required to become an optimist is to have a goal and to practice it. The more you rehearse optimistic thoughts, the more 'natural' and 'engrained' they will become. With time they will be part of you, and you will have made yourself into an altogether different person."[3]

Setting goals, even very small ones, is one powerful way

3 Sonja Lyubomirsky, *The How of Happiness: A Practical Guide to Getting the Life You Want* (London: Piatkus, 2010).

to actively build positive results into our lives. Another way that I found to be especially helpful for nurses is through the process of journaling. Gratitude journaling can be as simple as listing three people, places, or events at the end of each day or shift that we feel grateful for or with which we had a positive experience. This helps us recognize the highlights of the day that we might otherwise overlook. It's easy to forget about the one patient that said, "Thank you," when the other five yelled cuss words! But in taking time to remember and document these moments, we'll soon find there are more of them in the day than we often retain. Dialogue journaling is another great way to reflect on conversations that we have with patients or colleagues and to rephrase our potential responses for the next similar encounter. When we write down our negative response to someone, we can then rewrite how we would want to respond differently next time. In doing so, we give our brain different, more positive, alternatives to choose next time.

One example of active optimism is from travel nurses and nurses who have been reassigned due to changes in their facility in the last couple of years. A nurse can choose to do his/her best in whatever situation or unit they find themselves on any given day and set the tone for a positive experience.

Enjoy Smiles & Snacks

I started my nursing care in pediatrics, and it was such a rewarding specialty. No matter how sick or sad those kids were, they were always thinking about the next good thing. It might have been as simple as a popsicle after an IV start or bubbles after medicine, it didn't take much to get them smiling again.

I remember patients who would refuse to get out of bed for a bath or physical therapy, but would jump up and drag their IV pole down the hall and ride the elevator three floors down just to go visit the therapy dogs!

Pediatric patients are also really great at showing us how to think of others. Kids are always asking for craft supplies to make something special for their parents and extra snacks to share with siblings. While we are focused on getting *them* to feel better, they are often focused on making people around them smile.

Whenever I feel sad or overwhelmed with work or life circumstances, I think about how one of my patients would react. I try to think of something that makes me happy or brings me joy, even if it's just a yummy snack or good music. We can really learn a lot from kids about how to move past what hurts us and focus on what's fun, happy, and feels good.

Plan Self-Care

I had been a Med-Surg nurse in my local hospital for 5 years when I first felt the strain of my nursing career start to spill over into my personal life and personality. I became a nurse originally because my mom was a nurse and she loved her job, so I followed in her footsteps. She always found joy in her work and loved making a difference for her patients.

Just like my mom, I love interacting with my patients and seeing the positive impact I make in caring for them, but there have been a lot more deaths in the past 2 years than I was used to.

I started struggling to stay positive when I'd always been a positive person in my life before. Even when the pandemic first hit, people were cheering nurses on, clapping for us on our way into the hospital, and I felt powerful, like I could really make a difference for people. I felt like I could just hunker down and go to war against COVID because the whole world was supporting me. But after a while, people stopped being so supportive, and the pandemic dragged on. I started to feel like it would never end.

I tried to cope by eating comfort foods and sleeping in on my days off. I also tried to stay away from Social Media because of all the negativity. But I still felt overwhelmed.

With the help of The Resilient Nurse Project, I developed a better plan for self-care. I learned to moderate my comfort foods so that I could still enjoy them without harm and stopped feeling guilty about sleeping in. I realized that that was exactly what my mind and body needed during this stressful time. I started a simple exercise plan to lift my mood too!

Grab Your Notebook

I wanted to create a way to encourage my coworkers, so I put together an "Active Optimism" box for the breakroom. I included blank notebooks, stickers, and pens. People could choose a notebook and decorate it with the stickers, then use it to make a positive journal, listing things that happened in the day that were positive, or things they were grateful for. Sometimes we fill them out together at lunch. It's really helped people remember to think about positive things in the day, and talking about it together helps us have a more positive attitude on the unit instead of always negative. In a way, it holds us accountable for our attitudes and how we impact each other.

At one of The Resilient Nurse Virtual Summits, I learned that the World Health Organization says one of the signs of burnout is being cynical and negative. I told my colleagues this, and now every time someone says something negative, we laugh and say "grab your notebook!" It's a fun way for us to recognize negative attitudes and support each other instead of just getting dragged into the negativity.

Find Support

Working as a critical care nurse during the pandemic was the most challenging time in my nursing career. The isolation and the physical separation from family, friends, communities, and the activities that added more enjoyment to my life were emotionally challenging. I converted to being more of an introvert. My connection to God and my higher power and the support of my family, friends, and virtual communities had helped me through the tough times. I'm also blessed to be working with an amazing group of nurses, doctors, PCTs, NAs, leadership, etc. in one of the top hospitals in the nation. I couldn't think of a better place to be where they support the importance of wellness and mental health for their employees. I'm also part of several communities and coaching groups that were supportive as well as helping me with my personal and professional development for my nursing career and for my business. I was burnt out when I started to have a harder time sleeping at night and feeling disconnected. I started more yoga, continued my energy work, Healing Touch, and did a lot of meditation to help settle my mind and to help with my emotions.

I was able to use this time to do deep inner work of healing from trauma, emotional pain, etc. to transform my inner world so that I can make an impact in other people's lives: family, friends, patients, nurses, etc. This journey has led me to be a health and life coach to help others navigate the challenges that our world faces today. I'm so forever grateful for the support that I had that I would want to go beyond the walls of healthcare institutions to transform people's lives. So far I was able to make a positive impact with the help and support of my leadership and the nurses, doctors, PCT NA chaplains in transforming the human experience at the end of life as Chair of the MICU Palliative and Family-Centered Care committee. I also love working with my clients as I helped with self-care and as a health and life coach.

Vivien Joy Lamadrid

DECISIVE ACTION

"Knowing is not enough; we must apply. Willing is not enough; we must do."

— Johann Wolfgang von Goethe[4]

"Even if you are on the right track, you'll get run over if you just sit there."

— Will Roger[5]

"For as the body without the spirit is dead, so faith without works is dead also."

James 2:26

4 Xplore. (n.d.). *Johann Wolfgang von Goethe quotes*. BrainyQuote. Retrieved February 20, 2022, from https://www.brainyquote.com/quotes/johann_wolfgang_von_goeth_161315#:~:text=Johann%20Wolfgang%20von%20Goethe%20Quotes&text=Knowing%20is%20not%20enough%3B%20we%20must%20apply.,not%20enough%3B%20we%20must%20do.
5 Goodreads. (n.d.). *Will Rogers Quotes*. Goodreads. Retrieved February 20, 2022, from https://www.goodreads.com/quotes/23961-even-if-you-are-on-the-right-track-you-ll-get#:~:text=Quotes%20%3E%20Quotable%20Quote-,%E2%80%9CEven%20if%20you%20are%20on%20the%20right%20track%2C%20you',if%20you%20just%20sit%20there.%E2%80%9D

*"The wise prevail through great power, and those
who have knowledge muster their strength."*

Proverbs 24:5

What do a German poet, American humorist, and the Bible have in common? They all demonstrate the idea that knowledge, without action, is insufficient. Author Francis Bacon wrote that "knowledge is power."[6] When we choose to increase our knowledge, we have the power to *decide* the best *action* to take in the face of adversity.

Do you remember the first time you saw a patient in cardiac arrest? You might have frozen in fear or shook with the rush of adrenaline, but most likely, the experienced staff around you immediately began to follow protocols. Someone started compressions, someone worked on ventilation, and someone gave medications. Maybe the patient survived, or maybe they didn't. But what if no one took action? What if everyone just stood there? What if the doctors and nurses shared their knowledge about how to intervene but didn't decide to take action?

Stepping up and taking the lead in a code or crisis is a critical skill for nurses, and many fear they won't have what it takes to rise to the occasion when the time comes. Combine that fear with the trauma of witnessing a life-threatening event, comforting the patient's family members, and dealing with your own emotional response, and you may find yourself feeling completely helpless. According to Everly, Strouse, and McCormack, "The most powerful way of helping yourself in the wake of adversity appears to be resisting the pressures of psychological avoidance

---

6 Bartlett, John, comp. *Familiar Quotations,* 10th ed, rev. and enl. by Nathan Haskell Dole. Boston: Little, Brown, 1919; Bartleby.com, 2000. www.bartleby.com/100/. [31 February 2022].

and paralysis by doing something to help yourself or others. Take action."[7] Decide to do something, even if that something is handing over saline flushes. When the crisis is over, take time to review the event with a mentor or colleague so that you can increase your knowledge base for the next time and thereby increase your ability to determine and take the best actions.

Beyond what we learn in nursing school, there is so much more to discover through continuing education and specialty certifications. We can expand the catalog of information in our brain from which we can pull when decisions need to be made quickly. This knowledge building leads to becoming an expert in a chosen specialty or field. Many people choose nursing because of the variety of options, so explore those! When we can confidently make decisions, even if the outcome isn't what we wanted, we avoid the guilt that many nurses feel in questioning themselves after a situation is resolved.

---

7 Everly, Strouse, and McCormack, *Stronger*.

Decide How

Growing up, I loved to read, write, and touch books. To this day, I have stacks of books "to be read" all over my house, screenshots of recommended books on my phone... I just can't get enough! I thought about being a lot of things when I was young, and a book editor was on the top of that list. But life circumstances changed, and at the age of 20, I found myself as a young mom, facing divorce and another baby on the way. My dad sat me down one night while I was wallowing in self-pity and told me that, while I can't always choose IF I have to face a hard challenge, I can always choose HOW I face it. Those words awakened something new in me. At that moment, I realized how much I could change a situation if I just took action rather than sitting and waiting for things to happen. Those words have guided me through so many tough situations in the last 20 years. They led me to choose nursing as my career path so that I could provide security for myself and my children. They guided me as I watched my youngest child battle cancer at nine years old. And those words led me toward creating The Resilient Nurse Project.

Instead of just accepting the struggles of life and going through the motions in despair, I DECIDED to DO something about the situation. I researched resilience. I talked to other nurses. I listened to mentors. I read a TON of personal development books. Then I implemented action steps that would make a difference.

The time has come for nurses to stand up and advocate for each other, for safe work environments, mental and physical well-being, and adequate compensation. We can not continue to serve endlessly without receiving support in return.

Take Action

My colleague and I created one of the first independent nursing practice freestanding offices in the United States. We did so because we saw the need for a gap in middle-class care. We offered an assistant to overwhelmed doctors' offices at the time. We also continued our full-time jobs at the hospital. We spent a lot of extra hours offering patient care to those who had been discharged. They needed home care as well as office visits for various reasons. We were even mentioned in the Congressional Record. It took a lot of resilience on our part to overcome the obstacles.

Karon Gibson

*Read Karon's full story in her book, *Nurses On Our Own*.

Step Up

I became a nurse because I liked the money nurses made and I always liked science in school. I also always liked babysitting and kids in general so I decided to work in a pediatric ER when I graduated. Now I've been a nurse for 15 years, and there are so many new responsibilities being placed on us. I feel like younger people are getting into health care and then not being good at it, because new nurses have less and less clinical practice in school, and hospital orientations are shorter. The nursing shortage is not new, I remember talking about it in school 15 years ago, but it seems to have gotten much worse over the last 3-4 years.

I tried taking on more work to make up the slack and tried to schedule my shifts with colleagues I've known for a while so I knew my workday wouldn't be too bad, but I just felt so out of control sometimes on my shifts. I even started to look for other jobs, but all my friends I talked to who worked in other places felt similar things, so it didn't seem like the grass would be greener somewhere else.

The Resilient Nurse Project coaching helped me step back and spend some time doing self-care, clarifying my true inner desires for my career, and also creating a time in my schedule to relax and not be in charge of anyone or anything. I didn't realize how much my brain needed that! After the time of coaching and reflection, learning more about myself and what I truly wanted, I realized that I was not giving myself enough credit for my experience and how far I'd come as a nurse. The Resilient Nurse Project helped me realize that I actually *wanted* to be a leader so I could help make a change and encourage and teach the newer nurses in a more impactful way. I didn't want to change *where* I worked, I just wanted to stay there and help improve it.

I decided to go back to school and get my master's degree in healthcare leadership so that I could learn how to make positive changes and lead others well. Then, I applied for a leadership job at my work, and I got the job! I've helped make changes to our new hire orientation program on our unit so that nurses are better prepared to take care of our patients and can be better teammates.

By deciding to step up and own my leadership responsibility as an experienced nurse I was able to advocate for a better work environment. Even though we still have challenges, I feel empowered to help things get better instead of just stressing about them all the time.

Learn to Lead

I was put in the position of being a charge nurse after only being a nurse for two years. As crazy as it sounds, I was the most experienced nurse because so many nurses had left our unit after dealing with the pandemic for a while, they just didn't want to deal with it anymore. A lot of our nurses retired or moved to positions in an office with less stress.

I was still gaining confidence in my nursing skill, but I had never learned how to lead a team of other nurses or deal with angry family members. As long as the shift was going relatively normal, I felt comfortable being in charge. But I was always afraid that something would go wrong and I wouldn't know what to do at all.

In my coaching with Karen, I realized that I could learn leadership skills, how to de-escalate an angry visitor, and how to collaborate with other people in the hospital. Now, I know which patients to reassign when a new admission comes and how to replan staffing when someone calls out sick. I have built the skills and knowledge necessary to choose the best responses under pressure. Beyond my nursing skills, I learned how to lead, work with other non-nursing staff, and collaborate with other hospital teams.

MORAL COMPASS

Our faith, spiritual beliefs, and ethics, both personal and professional, are important parts of ourselves that we rely upon to help us make decisions and guide the care we give. Everly, Strouse, and McCormack suggest "that the moral compass for resilience consists of four points: honesty, integrity, fidelity, and ethical behavior."[8]

This concept of a moral compass comes to light prevalently in my conversations with Neonatal Intensive Care Unit (NICU) and end-of-life care nurses. When describing extreme measures for life preservation, they often tell me, "Just because we *can* doesn't mean we *should*." Balancing *quality* of life versus *quantity* of life is a difficult challenge for nurses, and relying on beliefs and values can help support our work when ethical questions arise.

This focus beyond the physical needs of our patients is often what sets nursing apart from other medical professionals. We do more than give medicine and perform procedures. We CARE for the patients. We comfort, we listen, we bathe, and we pray with them. Our ability to draw on our moral compass is a key factor in the holistic nature of caring for human beings. Learning to

---

8 Everly, Strouse, and McCormack, *Stronger.*

see death as part of the cycle of life is valuable when interacting with patients and their families.

Nurses also have the opportunity to incorporate the patient's values, beliefs, and practices like no one else because we spend so much time at their bedside. We understand how their morals impact their healing and hope, which can be powerful factors in their recovery or overall wellbeing. A moral compass is the "guiding light"[9] of resilience and decision-making.

9 Ibid.

Firm in Faith

As a pediatric ICU nurse, I spent many nights taking care of children who were victims of tragic circumstances. People often asked me how I could do the job, and my answer was always, "God." My faith in God gave me hope in even the darkest times. I felt honored to be the physical representation of His healing hands for the children, to comfort them and help them get well. I was thankful that God allowed me to provide compassion to parents as they dealt with worry, and reassurance when they felt unjustified guilt for a trauma they could not have prevented.

One particularly challenging group of patients to care for was victims of abuse. Many times, while police and social workers were investigating, we as nurses had to interact with the abusers themselves. I had to rely on my faith and integrity to show respect and not judge, even when I felt certain I knew the truth. My trust in God and His role as the ultimate judge allowed me to just focus on caring for my patient and being kind to everyone I encountered in the process.

Another really difficult part of being a pediatric ICU nurse is dealing with the loss of a patient. When a patient died, I had to focus on the comfort that I could provide in the process, and the dignity I could bring to the patient's end of life. I also created ways that I could personally honor those patients and process my grief in experiencing their death.

Stand Up for Yourself

Nursing requires teamwork. In each field of nursing I've worked, there was a team approach. The idea is to support and encourage one another and simply help each other. Someone needs to have your back. The importance of this cannot be emphasized enough.

My time at a health department was no different. I served in several departments there. Secure with 20 years on staff, a good salary, and benefits, I was sure I would stay until retirement. God had other plans.

I enjoyed the responsibilities of my last position with confidence, but the "team" part was lacking. We had good team members but no leadership. Communication was lacking and difficult to obtain. I was lucky to finish a question or sentence before they would abruptly turn and walk away. This was sadly well-known by many staff members.

It was an extremely uncomfortable situation. We dealt with county-wide, news-worthy health issues and I was on the firing line at times. I felt vulnerable and considered leaving (feeling that nudge from God) but clung to the security of salary and benefits. I was too scared to let go.

I hung on as it worsened. We became involved in a multi-county outbreak. The pressure was on. Our building became a command center, receiving all phone calls and responding to people who were sick and scared. I was totally overwhelmed trying to handle hundreds of calls and categorize them as contacts or newly diagnosed patients. I had lost weight due to the stress and long shifts, working overtime. I approached the team leader and told them I was struggling. They slammed down a stack of papers and told me, "GO

HOME!" I was shocked! There were others in the room. You could have knocked me over with a feather, as they say.

I left immediately, sobbing. When I arrived home, I penned my resignation and told God, "OK, I'm listening." Why hadn't I listened before? He had nudged me but this time He knocked me off my feet.

I turned in my notice the next day, with no emotion or question from my boss. On my last day, I requested just 5 minutes of their time. I could have filed a grievance but chose not to. I explained why I resigned and it was not taken well. I wanted to be done with this place. Before I left the office I said, "I'll pray for you." That wasn't taken well either.

I never regretted my decision and never looked back. Within a few days, my kids told me they noticed such a change in me. I seemed like a different person. The stress was gone.

Now, what was I going to do? I had to work. But who wants a 50-year-old nurse? New stress! Well, the following week 3 offers came to me without my searching. (That was God again.) A friend had been trying to recruit me to her office at UT student health. Why didn't I listen the first time!? Money!

I stayed 10 1/2 years and retired. It was an amazing experience and I made lifelong friends. We worked together! I was able to pray with students and staff. I have been so blessed!

I pray for this person regularly because they were so lost. I cannot hold a grudge.

Courage to Care

My last 10 years of nursing were spent at a university student health center. Best 10 years of my career! Some of us would tease that it is the largest pediatric office in the county. It truly is - the students are just big kids trying to find their way in the world. Many still need parental advice while others just need a hug and to know you care.

This was a time of growth for the LGBTQ community. Young adults were struggling with their identity. Our clinic was approved to offer hormone therapy for those wishing to change. I was uncomfortable actually giving the shots but had no problem caring for the patients themselves. It took a lot of courage for me to express this but I did it. Everyone involved accepted my position. It was a touchy subject.

To gain understanding and be efficient in caring for these individuals, I attended a conference in North Carolina regarding transgender issues and subjects, the gay community, etc. In a small group, I was singled out with the question, "How do you feel, as a nurse, about LGBTQ?" WHOA!

Hot, red face, sweaty palms, and tachycardia - I took a leap of faith. I said, "Well, I'm a Southern Baptist born and raised." He said, "Well then, what are you doing here!?" That got a laugh from all of us and helped me relax. I replied, "I believe the Bible, and the Bible says it's wrong. However, I'm a nurse and I will care for all my patients with the same respect and attention."

I was actually applauded. After the session, a man (dressed as a female) came over to me and said that he respected what I said (and also liked my outfit). I thanked him and went outside for some air.

I don't know where that courage came from other than God. The more you use your faith, the easier it is the next time. It's taken me a long time to learn that - to trust. But it really works!

Faith Foundations

I became a Christian at a young age. I grew up in church and my parents always tried to put our faith and beliefs at the center of our lives. For me, the Bible is the foundation of my moral compass. I try to live every day by what the Bible says, and do everything in a way that pleases God.

Because of my faith, I believe that everyone should be treated with kindness and love. I believe in miracles. I believe that God gave humans knowledge and wisdom to perform healing procedures and discover medications, but I also believe that He has ultimate power over everything we do.

When a patient has a positive outcome, I praise God for the healing. When a patient receives a scary diagnosis, I comfort and pray for them. Even when I don't understand why something happens, I am at peace knowing that God is in control in the end, and as long as my heart's intent is pure, He will honor my work. I am thankful that as a nurse I have the opportunity every day to show God's love to people.

RELENTLESS TENACITY

Many nurses find themselves in situations where they seek to change or improve a work process. These nurses also often find that changes are hard to implement when a manager or administrators are reluctant. We must not relinquish our ideas or our belief in improvement. However, some situations might require a creative approach or alternative way of communicating the justification and implications. Relentless tenacity applies in these scenarios because the change we desire might require multiple attempts or methods of introducing the idea to our administrators before we receive a positive response. If we're passionate about change in our unit that we believe is for the better, we shouldn't give up.

Relentless tenacity is critical now, with the increasing crisis of short-staffed, overworked nurses. An important element of relentless tenacity is understanding the boundaries that dictate when to "be tough" and when it's safe to process our emotions (i.e., at the end of a year or season, a semester, or shift). We permit ourselves to approach changes or stressors within the confines of self-respect. This "stick-to-it-iveness," this refining by fire, can be achieved with a persistent positivity, rather than aggressive complaint.

People often ask, "Isn't there a point where trying and trying just to try is no longer beneficial?" The answer is, "Yes!" When we see that our efforts cause distress or strife, then it's time to pivot or re-evaluate our approach, even if our end goal stays the same.

When the COVID pandemic began in 2020, the nursing profession adopted a collective fighting spirit. We felt like warriors. But we're worn out now. We're tired, and the system is not changing. Without a comprehensive set of resilience tools, we feel at our wit's end. This pandemic is a perfect example of the need for relentless tenacity. We hunkered down. We put our heads down and practiced "try, try again." Now it's time to identify other approaches, practices, and workplace cultural norms to bear these challenging times and make healthy progress sustainable.

Go for the Goal

I can't remember *why* I made the decision, but I distinctly remember sitting in my senior English class in high school and saying to myself, "I'm going to get a master's degree." Since that day, I maintained the goal as I navigated graduation and into college and adulthood. When I graduated with my bachelor's degree in nursing, I wanted to get a few years' experience under my belt first. After 2 years, I chose to apply for a master's program in business administration, so that I could understand the administrative side of hospital systems. But, in my first semester, I got distracted by a handsome man and well, my grades reflected the distraction! Instead of signing up for another semester of classes, I said yes to a marriage proposal and moved to a new state. My master's goal was put on hold again.

Five years into our marriage, and seven years into my nursing career, I decided to take another shot at obtaining a master's degree. I was still following the business route because I had a growing desire to own a business of my own or to lead a business that employed nurses. But I was distracted yet again in my first semester, this time by my daughter's brain cancer diagnosis. My only goal became making sure she got every treatment, medication, and therapy possible to keep her alive.

Four years after her diagnosis, she was stable in remission. I decided to give my goal one last try. I know that God led the way through this long journey towards my dream of obtaining a master's degree, and He made the path clear in my third attempt. Business wasn't supposed to be my focus. Education was. I applied for a program with a focus on nursing education, and in 2019 I graduated with my Master of Science! The details changed, the path had twists and curves, but I refused to give up on my original goal.

Write Your Life Story

If you had known me back when I was a 13 turning 14-year-old teenage girl you would have never known about the drugs and the drinking I was involved in. I was on a path that was virtually leading nowhere, always showing up to school drunk or stoned (when I decided to show up). This part of my teenage life was covered up by the constant involvement in school sports and countless hours spent at the swimming pool training for the next swim competition while mainly maintaining my grades. I still don't know how I was able to do this knowing what I was involved in. Eventually, I would start to give up on all the sports and any academics that I did have for people who I thought were my friends. This was part of my life that my family mainly my parents never did know the full truth about and to this day they still don't this is mainly because I was an extremely smooth talker that I had everyone believing what I wanted this included mental health workers, shadows, RCMP and social workers (many of these people I met after numerous failed attempts of suicide which resulted in hospitalization on the acute care floor and a diagnosis of manic depressive disorder or what some most professionals call Bipolar.)(this is only part of that time of my life to which I am not proud of). I still remember my dad telling me at one point that I would "end up on the streets, in jail or in a morgue" If I continued the way I was going.

It wasn't until I got pregnant at 15 with my beautiful daughter that I started to straighten my life out. She was my angel that I still believe showed up when I needed her most. When I started my nursing journey I had a very dark past from drugs, alcohol, depression, suicidal thoughts, abusive relationships, and luckily no criminal record (I came very close many times) now with only a grade 9 education I was determined to become a nurse to help others and share my story.

At this point, I was 32 years old with 5 children (Alishia, Dalton, Wade, Brayden, and Dusty) and although I did not meet the qualifications for the nursing program, I wasn't going to let them stand in my way with the help of a pilot project I finished my Bio. English, and Math in 3 months. This was all while having 3 boys in multiple sports including 3 different divisions of hockey, a baby just over 1 year, and working 2 part-time jobs. I had many obstacles during nursing school which included a pregnancy (Derek was born during the summer of my first year Aug. 2nd I returned to school when it resumed Sept. 9th for our second year he was just over 1 month old and was only 3 months for my first clinical), the loss of very close loved ones (my grandma and my mother- in-law I had to leave for 8 weeks (for a clinical)only 2 weeks after she passed away I didn't even properly grieve until later down the road), spending time (1 week) in hospital with my second youngest with croup complications (missing a week in nursing school is like missing a month), an academic withdrawal (I kept failing the skill testing there was a lot that never expected me to go back yet succeed), having to leave my young family for weeks at a time (9 weeks) (again this was leaving a baby under a year, a toddler and 3 other kids at home my daughter was older.) (I am was very fortunate to have a very supportive spouse that took care of the boys when I was away, one of the hardest things was coming home to the youngest not recognizing me and taking almost 1 week for him to come to me even though we FaceTimed daily) this was all while still working, even when it came to my licensing exam I was in the hospital with a ruptured spleen and was only released days before writing (I was not willing to reschedule so I drove with my spouse the almost 3 hours to write even still having pain at times and On meds for my spleen)

Even after all the struggles, I completed my nursing program. I was 1 of 6 that completed it. We started with approx. 35 students. (I did not complete it with distinction or honors I barely made the pass but.. marks are not what makes an outstanding nurse)

Fast forward I now hold a permanent position as an LPN with Alberta Health Services working in ER/Day surgery, I work casual on the Acute care floor and fit staff for the N95's, I am also currently taking my perioperative nursing course and I just completed my BLS instructor course through the Heart and Stroke Foundation,

(I started with AHS as a dietary aide prior to becoming an HCA and then LPN)

This was all while maintaining my home, children and doing what most thought was impossible, especially for a grade 9 dropout who got pregnant at 15 and was involved in all the wrong things. I will say although I had my family (spouse, kids, mom/dad, sisters, and in-laws), some very special faculty, and close friends that supported me, I think it was the ones that never believed in me that pushed me even harder to succeed.

"When writing the story of your life, never let anyone else hold the pen." Harley Davidson

Crystal Girard, LPN

Dig Deep

I began presenting Healing Touch and Holistic Nursing to my peers well over 30-35 years ago. During that time, I experienced being ignored, ridiculed, judged, and feared. I often had to dig deep to NOT judge back or want them to be receptive to what I offered, or to react when they would tease me.

The other situation is the resilience required as a travel nurse in the last 8 years. Again, being resilient about how staff would treat me like I was stupid, or too old, or too strange with a holistic philosophy. And again having to dig deep within myself to be at peace with who they were and accept their way of being; yet stay true to myself.

Rita Kluny

Never Give Up

My daughter is the reason I chose to become a nurse, but she also taught me resilience.

In 2017 I took a huge leap and started nursing school, everything was going great until in 2018 when I had just started my actual nursing classes my daughter was admitted to the hospital with respiratory failure. I had spent two months juggling between the hospital, school, and a toddler at home until my daughter was finally released after having an emergency tracheostomy placed. From there I spent the next 2 years focusing on school and my kids and it finally paid off when I graduated in September of 2020 and took my boards in October and was finally able to call myself Courtney Moses RN, BSN.

Those three years were the hardest years of my life between the late-night study sessions, the times spent in and out of the hospital with my daughter, to the multiple times I asked myself if I could do this. It is now February 1st, 2022, my daughter is now 10 my youngest is 7 and I just celebrated my first anniversary as a nurse and looking forward to what is in store for the years to come.

Courtney Moses BSN, RN

INTERPERSONAL SUPPORT

Interpersonal support refers to our colleagues, family, and friends—the people we can rely on when "the going gets tough." These are the people that we can talk to, in good times and in bad. They help us stay strong. When we need a space to grieve or acknowledge our struggles or let our guard down, having a group of supportive people allows us to fully process our emotions.

Having people to rely on when we're feeling overwhelmed is important, so much so that Abraham Maslow placed social needs just above physiologic and safety in his hierarchy of needs.[10] After you have your food, water, shelter, and safety in place, people are the next priority. But there's more to this need for social contact. The *type* of social contact matters—*who* we're with and *what* they're focused on. It's important for us to be part of a like-minded community of people who care about us, understand our struggles, and have the same desire for change.

We created this "new normal" of minimizing our contact to necessity, and often that necessity comes with negatives. With a global pandemic like many people have never even imagined possible, rising political unrest, and ongoing racial divide, people

---

10 Saul Mcleod, Maslow's Hierarchy of Needs," Simply Psychology, December 29, 2020, https://www.simplypsychology.org'maslow.html.

are scared, stressed, and confused. Patients and their families are increasingly judgmental and less trusting of the care we provide.

When we have permission to be vulnerable with our circle of supporters, and provide them support in return, we build a community that is "characterized by robustness, adaptability, and the capacity for long-term sustainability."[11]

11 Everly, Strouse, and McCormack, *Stronger*.

Find Your Person

I'll never forget the time when I was a new PICU nurse and I lost my first patient. He was a little boy that was in a house fire. He was my first patient death and the same age as my children. My dad was a firefighter, so one of my biggest fears growing up was that something would happen to my dad in a fire, so all of my worst fears came together in this one patient. I had only been a nurse for a few months. My mom worked close by, and when I got off work I drove straight to her office and just cried. I let myself feel all the different emotions, and then once I had those emotions and let them out, I could process the thoughts in my head. "Did I do the right things and make the right decisions as a nurse?" "Wow, doing compressions was kinda cool in a weird way." I also had to deal with the emotions as a mom with the loss of a child and how that related to my children. Having someone who I could pour all of those thoughts and feelings out to allow me to process each of them and each part of that grief as it happened and I worked through it.

We need to make sure that the person we rely on has the bandwidth and is willing to care for us in this way because not everyone is equipped for this type of exposure. Sometimes other nurses aren't the best because they have their own trauma to work through and they need space to heal. Or maybe it's someone like your spouse who loves you dearly but is not in the medical field and doesn't want to be exposed to that level of extreme hurt. We have to be mindful that we don't cause more harm by sharing our stories with people who are prepared to deal with them.

Ask For Help

I have worked as a nurse in a pediatric ICU for 6 years. My biggest struggle is that my husband and family do not understand the challenges I face. I love my job because I love kids and science and being able to heal/fix problems, but we see a lot of child abuse and traumatic deaths in kids and it can be very intense sometimes.

My husband used to listen to all my stories when I came home from work, but after about a year, my husband didn't want to hear my stories anymore. I can't blame him, it's a lot to take in. He doesn't work in healthcare so it's a lot for him to grasp. Since then, I've just kept them to myself. But it started to weigh me down. I tried talking to coworkers but we would just tell the stories over and over and not talk about ways to deal with the trauma.

Working with The Resilient Nurse Project program helped me figure out what level of help I needed, and I ended up getting a therapist that I could talk to and process the trauma that I saw at work. I also started scheduling alone time and created a ritual for honoring the patients I lost. That helped me find closure with especially tough cases. I've also started journaling about work and just by writing things down, I can process my feelings and unload my brain.

Build a Team

I work in a department where teamwork is highly valued. During our shifts, we are uber-focused on performing scheduled procedures, managing inpatient load, and handling unexpected add-ons. We work well together, but we rarely have downtime to chat. A few years ago, one of our team leaders decided to implement team events outside of work so that we could build camaraderie and get to know each other better on a personal level

Every Monday a group of us go out to dinner. The group varies each week based on everyone's work schedule, but the Monday dinner is a standing event for whoever can make it! People bring husbands and kids, and we have a rule that we can talk about anything EXCEPT work. Getting to know each other better has made our teamwork stronger and improved our communication at work.

This year we started doing once-a-month pedicure outings. On the first Saturday of every month, we meet up at a local salon and relax together. Sometimes we chat, and sometimes we all put in headphones and do our own thing. But we are still *together*, and just being in the same space together doing something that is refreshing and relaxing helps us support each other more.

Understanding who people are outside of work helps us better communicate, understand each other's stressors, and support each other at work. I recommend everyone create regular events outside of work for their team. Not everyone will be able to come every time, but the routine allows people a safe space they can consistently count on when they need it.

Nurses are Family

Our nurse colleagues often become our greatest supporters, even when our stress is from something outside of work. Many of us refer to colleagues as "work wives" because we get to know each other so well! One time, when my children were young, I got a call from the school principal that my youngest child was in trouble, in danger of being expelled. My husband and I had been dealing with her behavior issues for over a year, and this was the last straw. I walked into my boss's office and broke down into tears.

She could have asked me to leave or said that I needed to focus on work. Instead, she got up out of her seat, came around her desk, and hugged me. She allowed me to cry and comforted me. Then she told me that she would be there for me as I dealt with the issue at hand.

I've heard people say that nursing is one of the most trusted professions. Not only do our patients trust us, but we also trust each other. We have each other's backs, at work, and in every facet of life. We are in each other's weddings, attend each other's births, share vacations, and pick up each other's shifts. Nurses are family!

INTENTIONAL SELF-CARE

Self-care is often what people think of first when the topic of resilience is mentioned. Self-care covers the basics—the bubble baths, pedicures, massages, taking alone time—that a lot of people disregard because they know it's not enough. But self-care is an important place to start. Unless we practice it *intentionally*, it isn't likely to happen at all.

We have to slow down, be still and quiet, and give our brain space to process all of the physical, emotional, and mental demands on us, whether at work or in balancing work and home. I often coach moms who juggle being a mom, wife, and nurse, and they have to learn to purposefully make time to care for themselves. They make everybody else's doctor appointments, dental cleanings, etc. but don't prioritize their own.

It's often said that nurses are the worst patients. We don't take care of ourselves or put the same priority on our own needs that we do on the needs of others. We must schedule that self-care in our calendar, even if the why or how changes. However we fill that time can vary depending on our individual needs, whatever fills our soul or restores us, but the intentional part is critical. It is important to schedule that time and make it a priority. We have to decide that we will create a life in which we make time for ourselves. We are worth it, and only then can we truly care for others.

What can you forego to make this room in your schedule? There is a common saying that "you can't pour from an empty cup." We don't have to wait until the cup is empty before refilling it. Staying busy might numb the pain, but it doesn't heal it. Eventually, we'll run out of steam and still be left with all of the obligations and responsibilities that we tried to avoid.

Get Away

One of my best experiences with intentional self-care came recently when I attended a Cozy Winter Yoga Retreat designed specifically for nurses. Led by Brittany Stoeckel, Nurse Practitioner, and Yoga Teacher, the retreat aimed to guide nurses through restorative yoga, reflect on the previous year, and set intentions and goals for the new year ahead.

This retreat afforded me the opportunity to travel to a new destination, which is something I love to do! The temperatures were in the negative numbers, which I've never felt before. I went for a walk in the snow and enjoyed a cup of hot coffee sitting by a cozy fire.

In addition to the fun and adventure, I was able to spend time with other nurses, sharing stories of trauma and joy, struggles, and rewards of our careers. We talked about how each of us copes with the unique characteristics of our specialties and gave each other advice and encouragement.

By putting this event on my calendar in advance, I demonstrated for my children that intentional self-care is important. I also gave myself time and space to focus on my own well-being, and I returned home feeling refreshed, restored, and ready to take on whatever life brought my way.

Mindfulness Moment

During the pandemic, meditation was one tool I started using to deal with my stress that came from working in the COVID unit at the hospital. I discovered nursing coaching and got to dive in a little deeper. I have since had beautiful opportunities to share these moments with others. One of these opportunities occurred when our hospital decided to put down new flooring. This was a big project that seemed to last forever. My unit is smack dab in the middle of the main hallways and was going to be in the midst of construction for most of the time.

On one of the Fridays I was working, it felt like the construction was in our laps. It was extremely noisy. Drills, hammers, call lights, and our yelling to hear one another to communicate. We started the day by taking a collective breath and working together to not go crazy. The noise weighed heavy on us and the patients. Halfway through the day, I felt overstimulated and unable to think, and I noticed my nurses struggling too. Our mental strength was running thin.

I decided we needed to reset, take a moment to be present, and collect ourselves. It was a rare moment, where all my nurses were at the station, so I offered a mindfulness moment. We all stepped in an empty room and closed the door to quiet the drilling. I asked my nurses to allow their bodies to relax and be in their most comfortable position. We all closed our eyes and focused on our breathing. I guided us through a progressive relaxation to help release our tension, invited each of us to think about our purpose as a nurse, and ended us on some positive affirmations.

It physically felt like a weight had been lifted off of us. Later, one of my nurses told me, that her eye had started twitching from all the chaos and stress, but after we did the mindfulness and calmed ourselves down, it stopped. This moment strengthened us individually and as a team, and helped us recover from the difficulties of the day.

I'm so grateful to have learned these powerful tools. I have felt and witnessed their benefits. They continue to help me reset and show up for each new challenge.

Jenie Bennett

Customized Self-Care

Ever since I was a little girl and my baby sister was in the NICU, I knew that I wanted to be a NICU nurse. Now, I've been a NICU nurse for 3 years working night shift, and I'm a mom of an infant and toddler of my own! I absolutely love my job, and I even like working night shift, but the difficult sleep schedule that comes with it, plus the unpredictable, ever-changing sleep schedules of my kids, leave me feeling tired all the time. I manage to get sleep in when I can, but it's hard for me to find time to exercise and stay healthy. My schedule changes too much to commit to exercise classes at a gym, and I don't know how to go in and do exercises on my own very well. Plus, I don't like leaving my kids in childcare since I'm already away from them when I'm working. I do try to eat healthy as much as I can.

Working with The Resilient Nurse Project coaching, I was able to acknowledge that my health plan is just as important as my patients' health care plans. We identified realistic goals that were adaptable to my changing schedule but still effective. I learned to find exercises that my kids could do with me or that I could do with them, like yoga, going for walks at the park, and dancing! I realized that it's ok if my exercise and fitness plan looks different than others because I'm still meeting my goal of being active without sacrificing time with my kids, which is so important to me.

Novice Nurse Transitions

I became a nurse during the height of the covid pandemic. I had worked at my hospital as a tech during nursing school, so I already knew the environment and the people that I would be working with as a nurse. But I never imagined the challenges that would come from moving into a different role in the same unit.

The increase in responsibility that I faced was overwhelming. Nurses have to be so independent and make decisions quickly, even if they don't have all the resources and people they need. Within six months, I started feeling burnout, and I knew I had to do something quickly in order to survive.

I found a nurse coach who helped me process the stress I was feeling, and learn ways to cope. She taught me how to advocate for myself and to find extra resources to build my skills and knowledge further.

I also signed up for the Resilient Nurse Box subscription, so each month I would automatically have something to support me in taking care of myself. The books in the box helped me learn and grow, and the other items in the box were fun and useful!

I already feel much more capable of handling the stress of my nursing career, and I feel like I can help other nurses too as I learn ways to cope with burnout, exhaustion, and the other struggles that come with being a nurse.

SBAR: NURSE EDITION

I conduct a weekly live training in our free Facebook group, and one of the series is called "SBAR Nurse Edition." SBAR (situation, background, assessment, recommendation) is a communication tool commonly used among healthcare professionals. In the weekly series, I break down struggles that real nurses face today based on stories submitted to me about their careers, lives, and the balance between the two. I look at those situations and their backgrounds and ask questions like "What led to this situation?" or "What are the contributing factors?". From there, I assess the situation, identify the coping tools that the nurses currently use, and determine ways in which the struggles are, or are not, addressed. Based on the answers to these questions and the six pillars of resilience, I make recommendations. These recommendations are to help these nurses deal with the situation in a more resilient way. I love this series because it uses real nurse stories with real nurse challenges.

Typically, when one nurse struggles, they're not alone. If other nurses can identify with a situation, then the knowledge and use of these recommendations provide hope and valuable ways to work through any challenge, as well as potentially improve the situation for many. Nursing has evolved into a career that often leads to endless burnout, but that is not what it was created to do. We as the voice of collective nurses can change that. Here at The Resilient Nurse Project, we give you the tools to be your own advocate and develop a foundation of holistic, comprehensive resilience that allows nurses to withstand challenges and make positive changes. In one training session, I had the opportunity to share a recent experience and how using the six foundational pillars of resilience allowed *me* to work through a stressful situation in a positive way.

Situation: Currently, I am a nurse entrepreneur running my business, The Resilient Nurse Project. An issue that I run into as a nurse coach is that there is no traditional "benefits package" when you're your own boss. When issues arise, I don't have paid time off, sick leave, or short-term/long-term disability to support time away from my job. A business owner can purchase supplemental benefits, but they aren't provided automatically.

As an employee, balancing benefits and a bank of paid time off with the needs of three kids, myself, and a spouse is a challenge. If my child develops an ear infection, and I take a week off to care for her, what happens when I develop a sinus infection the following week? I don't have enough sick leave to care for my family and also myself, do I? It is a struggle. Even when I worked for one of the nation's top hospital systems with a full-time benefits package, it was still a struggle because the reality is that they were in control. I was at their mercy. I could only be sick or on vacation for as much as they thought was appropriate. I understand that organizations have to employ some kind of mitigation, so people don't call out sick every other week and constantly go on vacation, but that is not what this is about. This is about the ability to be what we need to be and have plenty of support and tools when a potential crisis comes our way.

Background: In the introduction of this book, I shared that I became a nurse out of necessity more than passion. Now, fifteen years later, my situation shifted such that I could be more selective about the specialty of nursing in which I work. My financial situation is more secure, and my kids are older. Now I can choose how to use my nursing skills and knowledge, but that also comes with its own set of challenges. This shift in my career is positive in many ways, but as with all change, it has the potential for pitfalls and adjustments, which may not all support my forward momentum.

Assessment: The beginning of this year threw me into a bit of a whirlwind. My oldest daughter was hit in the head with a piece of equipment at a winterguard competition, resulting in a concussion, and then two days later, she broke her foot. She is away at college, so I had to help her navigate the necessary care (doctors' appointments, x-rays, prescriptions) over the phone. While I could have driven to see her, it was important not to, which I will explain why later on. I had to make sure she was okay, received the care that she needed, saw a physician, followed up with the treatment plan, and obtained her medications. Later that same week, my youngest daughter (with a history of brain cancer) started displaying symptoms of COVID. Due to her risk of quick deterioration, we quickly took action so we could stay ahead of the game and make sure that it did not lead to a more concerning health risk. Fortunately, she did not have COVID and recovered quickly, but I still had to prepare and enter "alert" mode for any potential crises.

Now while all of this could have caused me to panic, I was able to work through this series of problems. I absorbed and addressed each issue and moved forward, but everything all at once still shook me a bit.

The following week, I received a call from my doctor about some concerning test results that needed further follow-up testing. That call was immediately followed by news that an extended family member was being hospitalized with a potentially serious health concern. This is when I started to feel stressed, but only for a few minutes. I could have easily become overwhelmed with worry or anxiety about how to take time off work, continue to ensure my children were well, afford to travel out of town to help a family member in need, *and* pay for additional health tests for myself. Luckily, my six pillars of resilience were solid.

1. *Active optimism.* I reminded myself that regardless of the outcome of any of these scenarios, I would get through it the best that I could, and I had a strong support system to see me through.

2. *Decisive action.* In earlier, calmer times, when I was not experiencing stress, my husband and I decided to build financial stability. We studied Dave Ramsey's "Total Money Makeover"[12] and implemented his teachings into our lives. We decided together to gain the knowledge to improve our financial position so that we were no longer reliant on our companies or jobs but ourselves. We could support ourselves with greater flexibility in times of distress. I also built a resilience plan that allowed me to maintain balance and calm through challenges in a variety of ways.

3. *Moral compass.* I relied on my faith. I asked God for peace, wisdom, and patience. I prayed a lot during these times.

4. *Relentless tenacity.* I said to myself, "I will not be defeated. Whatever challenge I face, I have every tool I need to help me face it with strength and courage." I reminded myself of this every time I started to feel uneasy.

---

12 Ramsey, D. (2013). *The total money makeover: A proven plan for financial fitness.* Nelson Books, an imprint of Thomas Nelson.

5. *Interpersonal support.* I called on my support system. I told them that I needed to share my struggles so that they could give me a little more love and grace in the moment.

6. *Intentional self-care.* I stepped away from work and allowed myself to process all of my different emotions. I journaled about all the different thoughts in my head, which allowed me to review those thoughts more strategically so that I could respond to them positively.

Recommendation: Before I give my recommendations, I want to ask you some questions. Do you have a personal resilience plan? Have you built a cushion or safety zones so that when life goes awry, your world isn't turned upside down? Or even if it is, can you deal with it? You don't have to be the fixer of everything. Have you recognized that? Have you figured out how to separate what you need to be in control of and what you need to allow other people to be in control of (i.e., the kid who is away at college needs to learn how to provide her doctor with her insurance information or get to the emergency room when she doesn't have a car)?

For my family members out of town, I reminded myself that I am not the fixer of that situation. When and if they call and say, "I need you," then I will attend to what they need, to the best of my ability. In the meantime, when all I have is information, I simply need to serve in a supportive role but not try to take on the role of fixer.

Have you decided that your employer is not your primary caretaker? This is a big one because a lot of people rely on paid time off or long- and short-term disability, and while those are helpful, they also tie you to that company that puts you at their mercy. Have you decided to advocate for yourself so that you aren't at their mercy anymore? I recommend that you do that.

You can still work for the same employer without being solely reliant on them for support. I recommend that you gain the knowledge you need about financial security, time management, parenting skills, or whatever else that you need to better your situation. Gain the knowledge you need to move *yourself* into a leadership position over your life, not in a spiritual but a practical sense.

I no longer have to rely on my employer to *hopefully* be supportive if something goes wrong. I learned how to identify and implement backup options by gaining knowledge about financial security and other factors that kept me afloat while I dealt with my obligations, personal welfare, and a surge of struggles.

This is The Resilient Nurse Project's mission in action. Everything we teach about using the six pillars of resilience truly works. This scenario demonstrates that having the right resilience tools, when I face what we all face at times, does not derail me. Giant hurdles become tiny bumps in the road, and I am able to move forward without falling apart. Life throws us all curveballs, but if we use a variety of resilience pillars to deal with and catch those curveballs, we can press on with a positive attitude and a renewed sense of purpose and efficiency.

CONCLUSION

Building a foundation of six strong pillars of resilience doesn't mean that everything is always perfect, but allows you to deal with challenges and approach them without feeling overwhelmed because you can rely on these tools to guide you. The diversity of these strengths aids you in addressing the variety and severity of life's challenges, big and small.

I hope you can see through the stories shared in this book how these six pillars of resilience can apply to any of the day-to-day struggles that we endure. One of the most valuable lessons that my parents taught me was that even when I receive help, I still have to help myself. Otherwise, I will never improve my situation or myself.

Commit to helping yourself today. Build a foundation of resilience so strong that not even the fiercest storm can uproot you. You deserve to be more than a victim of your career. You are a Resilient Nurse!

GRATITUDE

First and foremost, I want to give special thanks to story contributors Jan Fowler, Crystal Girard, Rita Kluny, Vivien Joy Lamadrid, Courtney Moses, and the many nurses who chose to submit stories anonymously. I can't put into words the amount of gratitude I have for my family and the support they give me. My husband, Brian, listens to all my dreaming and crazy ideas and encourages me to pursue every single one. My girls, Audrey, Haley, and Lauren, put up with my late nights and long naps and have always been my cheerleaders. And of course, I have to thank Champy for endless snuggles and for alerting me to every person, vehicle, and burst of wind that comes near.

My parents taught me to put Christ first, family second, and education third and to approach every part of my life with 100% effort. They demonstrate selflessness, unconditional love, and service to others every day. They also taught me how to laugh, enjoy life as it comes, and "roll with the punches." To sum it up, they are amazing—the best parents anyone could ask for!

I've also had the support of my in-laws, my brother and his family, and many aunts, uncles, and cousins along my life's journey. Each one holds a special place in my heart, and I treasure all the memories we've made.

To my PRB team, you all are phenomenal. Heather, you

are my editor for life! Alyssa, Stefanie, and Gabrielle, thank you for all the hard work you contributed to this labor of love. Amanda, thank you for being my cheerleader and marketing guru. You are such a wealth of knowledge!

Morgan, thank you for believing in me from the day we met. You've believed in every dream and mentored me to grow in so many ways. We're taking over the world, baby!

Finally, to every nurse I've ever worked with, I'm so grateful for the lessons, support, and camaraderie. Where would we be without each other?

ABOUT
THE RESILIENT NURSE PROJECT

The mission of The Resilient Nurse Project is to help nurses recognize, address, and overcome burnout and compassion fatigue. We offer classes, virtual and in-person events, employer curriculum, and more! Visit **rnproject.org** to find the best resources for you.

TESTIMONIALS FOR
THE RESILIENT NURSE PROJECT

"I love, love, love Karen's strategies for building resilience! Her masterclass gave me so many ideas. She breaks things down into 6 pillars and then provides PRACTICAL ideas that any of us can incorporate into our daily life! The idea of developing resilience can seem overwhelming – but Karen makes it doable. All nurses would benefit from her class! Highly recommend!"

"This was so, so good! Thanks a million. I'm so excited to be a part of this nursing revolution, it is past overdue."

"That was great, thank you! I loved all the heartfelt words and flow. It was perfect."

"Definitely going to try this after I give birth!"

"Thank you. That was so insightful and I love your message!"

"I got my box yesterday and it was amazing!!"

"I love Karen Fowler Furr's resilient nurse teachings, super helpful!"

"I just want to say thank you for putting together a beautiful nurse box!"

"Love my gift box!! Enjoying every bit of it. Thank you so much."